WATER
WONDER
WORKS...

A Guide to Therapeutic Water Exercises to Manage Arthritis Pain, Strengthen Muscles and Improve Mobility

Marti C. Sprinkle

CCB Publishing
British Columbia, Canada

Water Wonder Works: A Guide to Therapeutic Water Exercises
to Manage Arthritis Pain, Strengthen Muscles and Improve Mobility

Copyright ©2013 by Marti C. Sprinkle
ISBN-13 978-1-77143-074-6
First Edition

Library and Archives Canada Cataloguing in Publication
Sprinkle, Marti C., 1944-, author
Water wonder works : a guide to therapeutic water exercises to manage arthritis pain,
strengthen muscles and improve mobility / by Marti C. Sprinkle. – First edition.
Includes bibliographical references.
Issued in print and electronic formats.
ISBN 978-1-77143-074-6 (pbk.).--ISBN 978-1-77143-75-3 (pdf)
Additional cataloguing data available from Library and Archives Canada

Photo credits: All photos contained herein are copyright Marti C. Sprinkle.
Cover design and section pages designed by: Susan Bateman @ Zuli Creative Inc. www.zulicreative.com

Disclaimer: SEE YOUR PHYSICIAN. Before beginning any exercise program or changing your physical activity patterns, you should always consult with your doctor or physician, particularly if you have been inactive, are overweight, or have or suspect any sort of medical condition that might be worsened by exercise. This book is about managing arthritis pain, strengthening muscles and improving mobility, not treating disease. Do not use this book in place of proper medical care. All health questions concerning yourself or anyone else, including those pertaining to the use of therapeutic water exercises to manage arthritis pain, strengthen muscles or improve mobility, must initially be addressed by your doctor or physician. The author or anyone and anything associated with the writing, production or distribution of this book assumes **ABSOLUTELY NO** liability to or for anyone who uses the information presented in this book. The reader or user of the information presented in this book assumes the entire responsibility and liability for his or her actions.

Extreme care has been taken by the author to ensure that all information presented in this book is accurate and up to date at the time of publishing. Neither the author nor the publisher can be held responsible for any errors or omissions. Additionally, neither is any liability assumed for damages resulting from the use of the information contained herein.

Publisher: CCB Publishing
     British Columbia, Canada
     www.ccbpublishing.com

ACKNOWLEDGEMENTS

Writing this book has been a real eye opener for me. Getting started was the most difficult part because I knew how to perform the exercises in the water. Setting the exercises on paper and explaining how to perform them was a different story. I am grateful to all those who eagerly and diligently encouraged me to write this book and to those who contributed invaluable knowledge and expertise.

I would like to thank all my many clients who kept asking me to write this book. They wanted something on paper that they could take with them when they traveled. Some of my clients even gave a name to an exercise.

Michael C. Loehrer, author and assistant pastor of Bear Valley Springs Church, encouraged me to write at least an hour per day. I didn't.

Eventually, I sat down and wrote for several hours at a time, conceiving exercises through from start to finish, which led to the completion of this book. My author friend and historian James Bullock gave me helpful suggestions and often advised me to visualize the finished book.

I would also like to express my gratitude to the Bear Valley Springs Association, a non-profit corporation governing the resort community located in Tehachapi, California. Debbie Papac, the Bear Valley Springs recreation manager, allowed me to initiate my Therapeutic Water Exercise program in the spa seven years ago. Neither of us knew how the community would react. The program had been approved by the Bear Valley Springs Association general manager, Kirk Woolridge, CMCA, CHA and the Board of Directors. Just last year, Debbie Papac asked me to extend the program.

The Therapeutic Water Exercise Classes at the spa are now full, thanks to the staff at the Whiting Recreational Center and the maintenance crew. My clients receive much desired attention and the spa is well maintained. My youngest client, this summer, was 8 years old, and my oldest is 92.

I am immensely grateful to Jay Sussell, my friend and client, for serving as a model for my second photo shoot. Thank you also to Darilyn Dickson for excellent photos as well as to Randy C. Horne of Picture This Graphics for my first photo shoot.

My friend Malissa Miller, EMT and Red Cross advisor, suggested that I use photos rather than sketches because they would be easier to understand. I am glad she did because the photos add a more professional look to the book and help readers.

My special friend and someone I consider an adopted daughter, Susan Bateman, helped me with the graphic design of the cover. Susan has her own business in San Diego -- Zuli Creative, Inc. She took time from her busy schedule to create the cover design of this book.

Dr. Wayne Wundrum, DC, a chiropractic specialist, helped me with some floor exercises, which I adapted to the water and have used for many years in all my classes.

Special thanks to all of my instructors from Aquatic Therapy and Rehabilitation Institute and American Exercise Association for teaching me many of the techniques which I use for my classes. Their classroom explanations and techniques inspired and encouraged me with the writing of this book. These instructors, including Sherlee Beebe, Laurie Denomme, Terri Mitchell, Beth Scalone, Maryanne Haggarty, and Pauline Ivens, along with many other wonderful instructors, continued to inspire me to provide more for my clients. The founder of both ATRI and AEA mentioned above, my friend Ruth Sova, a professional, has spurred me many times to write this book.

The help from my computer technician was wonderful. Alexander Kuntsmann spent countless hours formatting the graphics on each page. His assistance was essential to the completion of the final product.

Thanks to Dr. Roger Van Ommeren, Ph. D. in journalism who edited the manuscript.

SPECIAL ACKNOWLEDGEMENTS

With gratitude, I thank Dan Steinburg, Masters of Science, physical therapist of Stone Mountain Physical Therapy, for his invaluable help and encouragement with the muscle and muscles groups mentioned within this book. Stone Mountain Physical Therapy is located in Tehachapi, California.

Dan Steinburg is a graduate of the University of California San Francisco Medical Center and received an advanced degree from UCLA. He taught at the University of New York - Buffalo and also at Boston University. Dan has over 47 years of experience in the field of physical therapy.

Dan's guidance with the generalization of muscles/muscle groups for each exercise inspired me to continue the writing of this book. He felt that perhaps the book had professional merit as well. Dan's experience and expertise helped me to more fully comprehend the precision of each exercise presented.

PREFACE

The exercises described herein are intended
to relax muscles and ease movement while delivering
a soothing, stimulating low-impact workout. They are
to be performed only as instructed and at your own
risk. No medically endorsed therapeutic or curative
benefits are implied.

---

*"Ten years ago Relapsing-Remitting Multiple Sclerosis left me with
limited mobility. Muscle spasms and impaired muscle control
eventually led to my using a cane and an ankle-foot orthotic.
Desperate to find some type of activity, I turned to water therapy
and water aerobics as a means of gaining control over my body.
After 7 years of aquatic classes, I can now walk without a cane or
an ankle-foot orthotic. My range of motion, balance and cardio
health have improved my confidence, body tone, weight and overall
energy and health. Peace and blessing to anyone who becomes
involved with aquatics."* – Pat C.

TABLE OF CONTENTS

INTRODUCTION

Everyone wants to become healthy or to increase their range of motion as they age. Working individuals have limited time and attempt to increase their physical activity at home. The exercises presented in this book can become life-changing for you. These simple exercises, if performed regularly, will help improve how you feel physically and increase your feeling of well-being.

This book is designed to be used in your own hot tub or spa. Some of the exercises can even be done in a bathtub. All of them can be performed in a swimming pool, standing and/or squatting in shallow water. Many home spas do not have an upright bench, but a small plastic bench (or plastic chair) with a punctured tennis ball at the bottom of each leg to prevent scratching can be placed in the center of the spa so that the exercises can be completed as shown.

For individuals using a hot tub or spa at their home, the recommended water temperature for the exercises shown in this book should not exceed 94 degrees Fahrenheit. The recommended water temperature for therapeutic water exercises ranges between 88 and 92 degrees. For sports injuries or muscle problems the water temperature should be set towards the higher end of this range, but is not to exceed 94 degrees.

When doing a free body exercise, especially in water, it is difficult to determine which part or section of the body is involved because the whole body participates in the activity. Land exercises and weight machines isolate a muscle or muscle group. In water many more muscles become active with each and every exercise.

The exercises in this book are presented by sections of the body: Upper Body, which includes shoulders, Hands and Wrists, as well as the fingers, Lower Body, the Neck and some additional Upper Body Stretches. Each exercise has a title and a general direction followed by illustrations and the exact way to perform the exercise. The muscle groups noted under each set of photo images were identified by Dan Steinburg, physical therapist. Most of the muscles mentioned are the more important muscles upon which the exercise focuses.

The exercises in each section are grouped so that one can choose the exercise that suits whatever muscle appears to be stressed or aching from sports activities or from daily living. Individuals can experience restless sleep and awaken to find a muscle or muscle group is aggravating them. By selecting one or two exercises that target the area of stress or trauma, a person can relieve the pain by working out the muscle stress in the water.

To follow and complete all exercises presented in this book will take much more than an hour. This book is designed to serve as a personalized guide to individualize routines based upon muscle need. For example, one might choose Big Arm Circles, Flying or The W for arms and shoulders; then, move to Toe Point, Butterfly Knees, and Leg Lifts for the ankles, hips and knees, followed by "Piano," Thumbs Circles, and Thumb Stretches for the fingers; and conclude with Looking, Pendulum Neck Stretch, and Nods for the neck. After choosing several different exercises, one can develop a favorite routine to suit individual needs and add new exercises from this book to compose routines.

Relax and enjoy your water experience. You are only a few strokes away from feeling a whole and different you. Water has a most wonderful, amazing, and somewhat magical effect upon the human body. Water massages the body with an energizing effect almost like a caress.

1

UPPER BODY

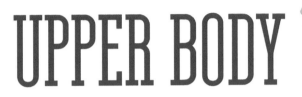

"I can work my muscles without pain. My posture has improved and I walk more upright." – Doreen I.

"The spa therapy exercises have been beneficial for toning and relaxing my muscles due to age related issues. I feel as if the circulation in my feet, legs and arms has improved." – Terri S.

"I am a diabetic who has poor circulation and arthritis. Water therapy has helped improve my health tremendously. Not only is my blood sugar down and stabilized, but my aches and pains are now minimal. Water therapy has been good for my mental status and self-esteem." – Judy A.

Big Arm Circles

Bring arms to the surface of the water, out to the sides as far as possible. Using both arms, bring the hands together in front of seated torso, circling arms toward the chest area, as if encircling a large balloon to squeeze out the air. Keeping the hands cupped and under the surface of the water, return the hands to original position. Repeat the exercise 12 times.

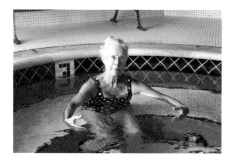

Arms are under the surface of the water, hands are cupped in a ready position.

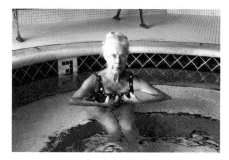

Arms are brought into the chest as the first repetition is completed. As the arms circle around and outward they should be fully extended below the surface of the water. Reverse the motion returning arms out to the sides.

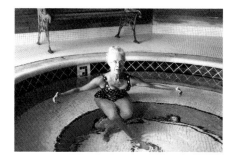

Arms are fully extended on the surface of the water. The exercise is repeated for 11 more intervals. It is then repeated as if performing the breast stroke.

The water buoyancy of this exercise assists with shoulder elevation. The posterior shoulder girdle muscles are strengthened. The Pectoralis major muscle groups are stretched. Upper shoulder mobility occurs.

Flying

Arms are placed on the surface of the water, out to the side, palms down. Keeping arms straight move them down and up as if flying. The arms should move down and up, 6 to 8 inches below the water's surface, to the lower rib cage area in the water. Repeat "flying" for 12 times. The exercise is repeated with palms up. Keep palms up and "flying" for 12 times.

To begin the exercise, arms are out to the side on the surface of the water, palms down.

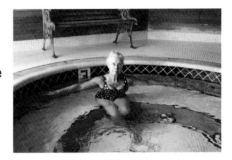

With palms down and arms straight out to the sides, move the arms down and up 6 to 8 inches, near the lower chest.

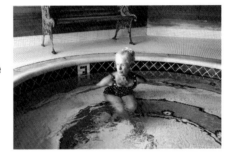

This photo shows the palms up as the exercise is repeated. The arms still move to the lower chest area and up to the water's surface.

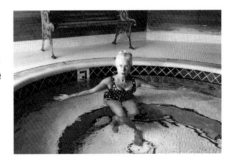

The subscapular and pectoral muscle groups are strengthened and stretched with this exercise. The buoyancy of the water helps arm elevation.

Circles

Keeping both arms straight out to the side with the palms up, make 3 sizes of circle rotations with hands and arms under water, using a forward motion (tennis ball, basketball, and beach-ball sized); then, reverse the arms rotations beginning with the largest sized circle, ending with the smallest sized circles. Repeat for a minimum of 12 times.

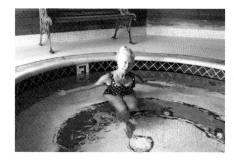

Arms are outstretched to the sides of torso, level with surface of the water and fairly even with the shoulders.

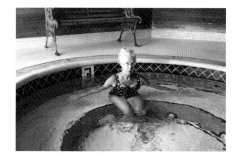

Palms are up in a ready position. Circle rotations begin. Palms stay up, but do not make circles below the hips. Each sized circle should be repeated for 12 times.

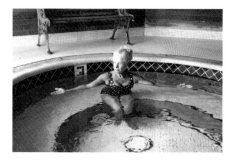

Arms remain extended at the sides of torso. Reverse the times of the above arm circles.

The posterior shoulder girdle and the pectoral muscle groups are strengthened and stretched with this exercise. The buoyancy of the water assists with shoulder elevation.

Clapping Hands

With both arms straight, clap both hands in front of torso. Then, separate and move the hands, palms out, to touch the wall of the hot tub behind the torso. Turn palms inward and bring palms back to the original clapping position. If possible, clap the hands in front and in back of torso for a full range of shoulder motion. The moving palms should be kept out while moving away and turned inward when moving back to the original clapping position. Repeat for a minimum of 12 claps.

Hands are held under the water's surface with palms together in an exercise ready position.

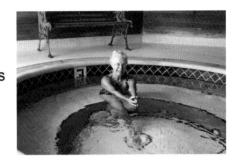

Arms are moved toward the back of the torso with palms out. Keep arms, with palms out, just below the water's surface, even with the shoulders.

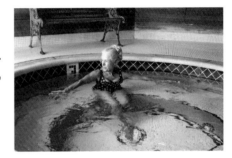

Arms are returned from touching the wall, or clapping behind the torso. Palms are turned inward and kept just below the surface of the water. Arms are returned to the original position clapping in front of torso.

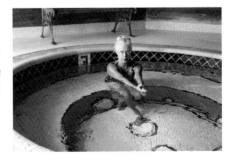

The clapping of the hands works the Pectoralis major muscle groups. Clapping behind the torso or as close as possible to clapping behind the torso works the middle Trapezius muscles, the Rhomboid muscles, the posterior Deltoids, the Teres major, and the Infraspinatus muscles.

Upper Torso Stretch Using Clapping Hands

Clasp palms together in front of torso just below the water's surface. Move clasped hands from side to side, from shoulder to shoulder. To extend the benefit of this exercise, move clasped palms to the right looking over the left shoulder. Then, move clasped hands to the left side looking over the right shoulder.

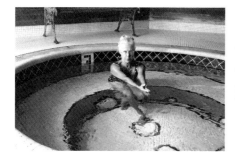

The hands are clasped together in front of torso just below the surface of the water and even with the shoulders. The palms of the hands are together.

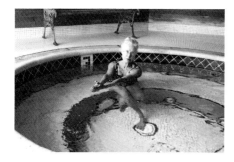

Both arms move to the right. The arms are at shoulder height. The head and chin turn to the left as the arms move to the right. The palms of the hands are together. Both arms move to the left (not shown). The arms are at shoulder height. The head and chin turn to the left as the arms move to the right.

This exercise works core muscles plus alternating the external/internal obliques with the Multifidus and Erector spinae. The abdominal obliques are turning the torso in cooperation with spinal muscles on the same side of the torso. Turning right stretches the posterior shoulder girdle muscles and strengthens the Pectoralis major. Turning left reverses the effect on the left and right posterior shoulder muscles --- Supraspinatus, Infraspinates, middle Trapezius, and lower Trapezius.

Rowing

Stretch arms out in front of torso on the surface of the water. With palms down, make a fist. Then, make a rowing motion with the fisted hands, bending the elbows to make a circular motion by the side of the torso. Make sure the elbows come back far enough to pinch the shoulder blades together. Row forward 12 times. Then, reverse direction and row backwards 12 times.

Arms are extended in front of torso below the surface of the water and even with the shoulders. Palms are closed into a fist.

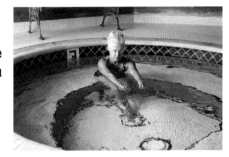

The fisted arms "row" forward over the surface of the water. Elbows are bent as the fisted hands come over the surface of the water, down toward the hips, circling, and returning to the start position.

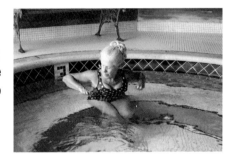

This photo depicts the placement of the fisted hands as they "row" around the back of the hips to complete the circular motion. The arms complete the circle and extend out in front of the torso for each repetition.

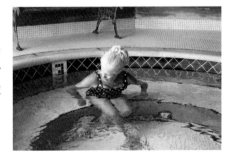

The exercise is repeated in the reverse direction, or a backwards "row." When the exercise is completed, forward and backwards rowing, the arms should return to the surface of the water.

The water buoyancy of this exercise helps shoulder elevation. The water's resistance helps strengthen the posterior shoulder girdle. The stretching assists the Pectoralis muscle group.

Pull-Push

Place the arms straight out in front of torso so they are even with the shoulders and on the surface of the water. Keep palms open and facing down. "Pull" the flat palms down to the hips, or as close as possible. At the hip level, turn palms up and "push" the water to the surface. Repeat this exercise for 12 times or as often as is comfortable. Increase attempted times each time the exercise is performed until a minimum of 12 times is achieved.

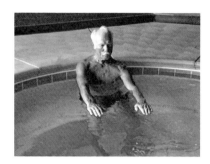

Flat palms are placed on the water's surface in front of the torso.

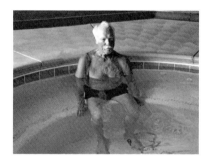

The palms are pulled downward near the hips.

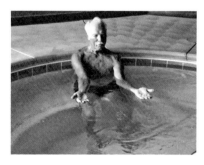

With the flat palms turned upward, push the water upward, causing the palms to return to their original position. This push/pull motion is repeated for 12 times.

The upward movement of this exercise strengthens the Pectoralis muscles; the downward movement strengthens the Latissimus dorsi muscles. The water's buoyancy assists shoulder elevation.

Alternate Hip-Palm Pull

Arms are extended straight out in front of torso on water's surface. Palms are flat, facing down. "Pull" right palm and across the torso to left hip keeping the arm as straight as possible until it passes the middle of the torso. Then, bend the elbow and touch the hip. Return flat palm to starting position. Repeat the movement, pulling the left palm to right hip. Alternate the arms, right/left, keeping palms flat, counting each alternating move as one repetition. Repeat for a minimum of 12 times.

Flat palms are extended out in front of the torso on the water's surface.

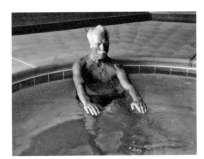

The right flat palm is "pulled" across the torso to the left hip. The arm is kept as straight as possible until it passes the mid-torso area. Then, the flat right palm "pushes" the water to return to the water's surface.

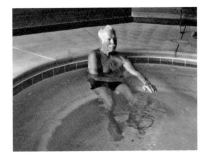

The left flat palm is "pulled" across the torso to the right hip. The arm is kept as straight as possible until it passes the mid-torso area. Then, the flat left palm "pushes" the water to return to the water's surface.

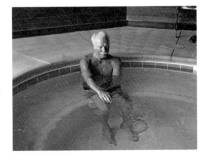

The stretching movement of this exercise helps strengthen the Erector spinae and abdominal oblique muscles. The rotational movement in this particular exercise would be most helpful to someone with Parkinson's disease.

Elbow Bends

Float the arms on the surface of the water with flat palms facing the bottom of the pool. Bend the elbows and pull the arms back even with the shoulders, keeping palms flat. Pull the flat palms down. Then, bring the hands back to the surface of the water. Keep the upper arms from the shoulder to the elbow on the surface of the water with palms down. Repeat the exercise 12 times always bringing the flat palms to the water's surface.

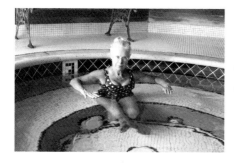

The upper arms are floating on the surface of the water even with the shoulders. The palms are flat.

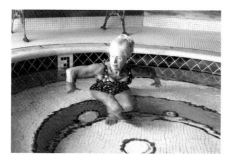

Flat palms are pulled downward. Return the hands to the water's surface. Repeat 12 times.

The water's buoyancy is stretching and strengthening the internal rotators of the shoulders, the Subscapularis muscles (as shown in first photo above).

Elbow "Flaps"

Float bent arms on the water's surface, palms down and forming a 90-degree angle at the elbows. Pull the bent elbows to the sides of torso. The palms will come together. Then, pull the elbows up/down to the water's surface, like "flapping wings" or as if playing an accordion. Repeat this "flapping" 12 times.

Elbows are bent at a 90-degree angle and arms are floating on the water's surface.

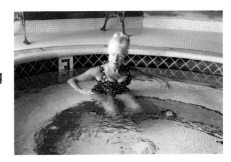

Elbows are pulled down to the sides of the torso. Palms of the hands face one another. Fingertips remain together.

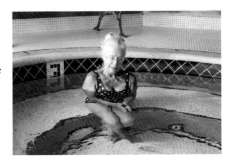

Elbows are brought back to the surface after touching the rib cage. This puts the elbows back to the starting position and ready to begin another repetition.

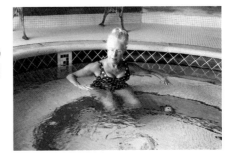

This exercise strengthens the Latissimus dorsi and the Teres major muscles groups.

Fixed Elbows

Keep bent elbows at your sides with the forearms extended in front and the palms flat in a clapping position. Move only the flat palms and forearms apart and together in front of the torso without moving the elbows from their position on the rib cage. Pretend the elbows are glued to the rib cage. Continue moving the flat palms back and forth through a minimum of 12 times.

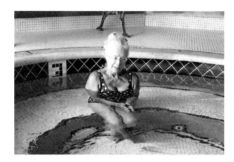

Elbows are at the sides, like keeping them stuck to the rib cage. The palms are facing inward, and the arms are extended in front of the torso and in line with the elbows. The bent elbows rest at a 90-degree angle.

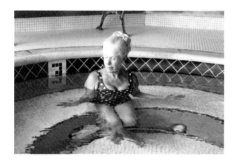

The elbows remain at the rib cage. The flat palms go out to the side as far as possible without moving elbows from the side of the rib cage.

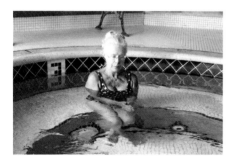

The elbows remain at the rib cage. The flat palms come back into the front of the torso touching lightly before the palms go back outward like a seal clapping its flippers.

This exercise will strengthen the Infraspinatus and the Teres major muscles.

Elbow Extensions and Flexion

Float hands on the water's surface with bent elbows, and finger tips together in front of the chest. The palms remain flat. The elbows drop, rotate or move downward, and in toward the torso, lower chest area; then, outward away from the chest/torso area. Repeat for 12 times.

Palms are flat and fingertips are together, touching, and in front of torso. The elbows are raised even with the shoulders as flat palms, fingertips together, float and rest on the water's surface.

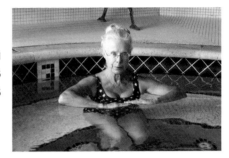

The elbows rotate inward toward the torso, lower chest.

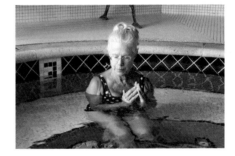

After touching the torso, the elbows are pulled upward and brought back to the water's surface, keeping them as even with the shoulders as possible.

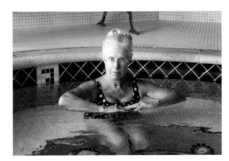

This exercise flexes and extends the elbow joints. The resistance of the water helps strengthen the Triceps and stabilize the elbow. The arm flexions strengthen the Biceps.

Swimmer Arms (Arm Stretches)

Float arms with bent elbows on the water's surface. Extend one arm on the water's surface keeping flat palms. Alternate the arms as if performing a swimming stroke. Stretch each arm as far forward as possible without raising the torso. This exercise should be repeated so that each alternating arm performs 12 times.

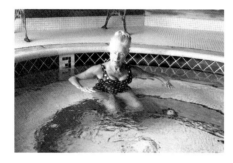

Arms with bent elbows are floating on the water's surface. The arms are shoulder height and the elbows remain at shoulder height as well.

Photo 1: If the arms are buoyant, there is no muscle action. If the arms are not buoyant, the Deltoid muscles are utilized.

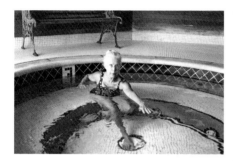

The right arm is stretched out in front as far as possible, keeping palms flat. The arm that remains in the original position is slightly pulled back so that the stretching arm can be extended as far as possible.

Photo 2: When the arm reaches forward, the anterior Serratus and anterior Deltoid muscles are used. When the arm reaches backward, the posterior Deltoid and middle Trapezius muscles are utilized.

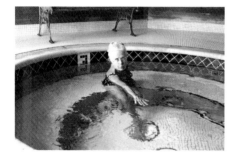

The left arm is stretched out in front as far as possible, keeping palms flat. The right arm has moved back and may be pulled slightly backwards to allow the left arm to stretch forward as far as possible.

Rotation of the spine requires external abdominal oblique muscles and internal abdominal oblique muscles to stretch and strengthen. The spinal Extensors will alternately contract and relax with the change of direction.

Hands Up

The hands are floating palms down with bent elbows on the water's surface. Begin the 12 times by raising the back of the hands until fingers point up. The elbows should point down toward the waist.

Start with palms downward and the arms floating on the water's surface. Hold the arms with bent elbows at shoulder height.

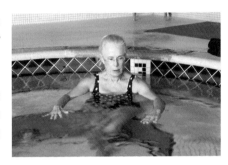

Photo 1: This part of the exercise is an isometric contraction of the muscles. The rotation upward activates the Supraspinatus, Teres major, and Infraspinatus in a concentric contraction.

The flat palms are rotated upward keeping the elbows bent. This gives the appearance of "hands up."

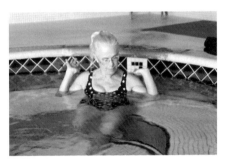

Photo 2: This "hands up" exercise is an eccentric movement of the muscles mentioned above.

The flat palms are once again brought down to the water's surface, keeping the elbows bent and the arms at shoulder height. Repeat this "hands up" for 12 times.
This "hands up" exercise is an eccentric

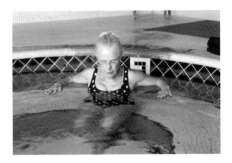

Photo 3: The exercise works the following muscles: Infraspinatus, Teres major, Rhomboid, and middle Trapezius. If the spine is erect and maintained erect throughout the exercise, then, this exercise becomes a back and shoulder exercise as well.

The W

The arms with elbows bent at a 90-degree angle are held at shoulder height on the water's surface. To perform the exercise properly, the spine is straight and the palms are flat, facing down. Move arms so hands point to the ceiling. The elbows with the upraised hands are firmly kept in place. Both elbows are then pulled backward simultaneously and then brought forward to the starting position. The head faces forward for spinal alignment. **Only** the arms with palms flat move forward and backwards. The exercise should be repeated 12 times.

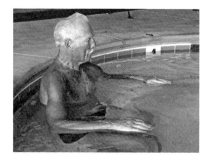

The arms with bent elbows are at shoulder height and on the water's surface.

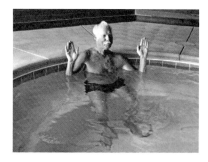

The flat palms move to point toward the ceiling. The elbows are kept bent and elevated.

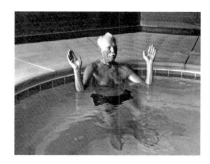

The elbows with bent arms are pulled backwards as if pinching the shoulder blades together. The elbows are brought forward after the spinal pinch.

Muscles groups worked with this part of the exercise are the Teres major, Infraspinatus, Teres minor, Rhomboid, and lower Trapezius. When the shoulder blades are moved backward, the middle Trapezius are contracting; when the shoulder blade moves forward, the Pectoralis major muscle is strengthened and/or challenged.

Push Up the World (Alternate Arm Stretches)

From the previous exercise, the arms are brought back to the "W" position. The elbows remain bent and the finger tips point up. The palm is pushing toward the sky/ceiling ending in a flat position as the arms are alternately raised and brought back downward to right/left W position. The flat palm is briefly held upward so that the side of the torso is stretched. This "Pushing Up the World" is repeated 12 times.

The right arm "pushes" the palm of the hand toward the sky/ceiling. The right palm ends up in a flattened position and is held there briefly to stretch the side torso.

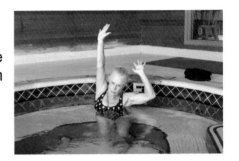

The left arm "pushes" the palm of the hand toward the sky/ceiling. The left palm ends up in a flattened position and is held there briefly to stretch the side torso.

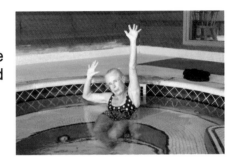

This exercise requires a progression of coordinated muscle action of the neck and scapular muscles.

Hold Up the World and Twist It

Continuing from the previous exercise of "**Push Up the World**," both arms are simultaneously pushed and held upward with flat palms for approximately 30 seconds. At the end of 30 seconds, the upper torso is turned first to the right and then to the left "twisting" the upper torso. This twisting movement is repeated for only 2 times on each side, right and left.

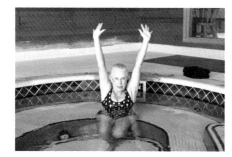

Both arms are pushed and held upward with palms flat, toward the sky/ceiling. This position is held for approximately 30 seconds.

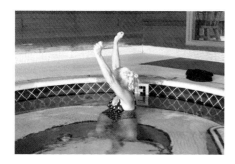

At the end of 30 seconds, the palms are turned first to the right and then to the left "twisting" the upper torso.

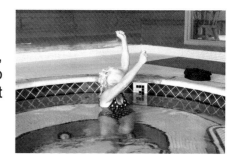

The reaching segment of this exercise "challenges" the Triceps, Supraspinatus, Deltoid, and Serratus anterior muscles. This stretch requires the use of the Latissimus dorsi, thoracic Intercostal muscles and the abdominals.

This exercise alternates the use of the external and internal olique abdominal muscles and stretches the Erector spinae.

Water Skier Arms

The arms are bent and held at waist level. Hands form fists. The fists are pushed out in front and then pulled back simultaneously. The fisted hands are brought backwards even with the rib cage at the same time. This push/pull of the arms should be repeated for 12 times to get the best results.

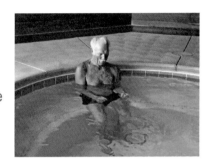

Arms are held by the sides of torso. Both hands are in a fist.

Photo 1: The Subscapularis, and Latissimus dorsi muscles are utilized at this step of the exercise.

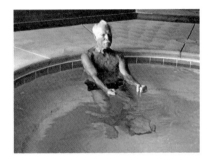

Fisted hands are pushed out in front and then strongly pulled back toward the torso. The elbows may pull beyond the torso/waist as the fisted hands are pulled backwards.

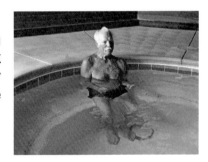

Photo 2 (directly above): With a forward push, the anterior Deltoid muscles are utilized; with a pull/push the posterior Deltoid muscles are utilized.

Underarm Swings

To begin this exercise, the arms are straight in front floating on the water's surface, palms down. The right arm is moved straight to the right side leaving the left arm straight with a flat palm. The right hand is fisted, and then with a swinging motion, the fisted palm is pulled under the straight left arm underneath the elbow. This movement is performed for 12 times. Then, the right arm is extended with flat palm in front of the torso. The left arm is moved to the left side. The palm is fisted, and then with a swinging motion, the fisted palm is pulled under the straight right arm underneath the elbow. This movement is performed 12 times.

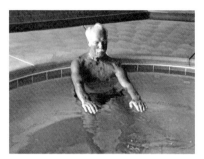

The arms with flat palms are floating on the water's surface.

Photo 1: If the arms are buoyant, there is no muscle action. If the arms are not buoyant, the anterior Deltoid muscles are utilized.

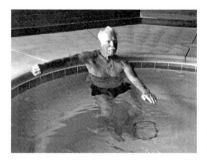

The right arm is moved to the right side leaving the left straight arm extended with a flat palm. The right palm is fisted. The arm is kept straight. With a swinging motion, the fisted palm is pulled under the straight left arm underneath the elbow. This movement is repeated 12 times.

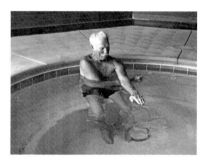

Photo 2 (directly above): The posterior Deltoid, middle Trapezius, Subscapularis, and Pectoralis major muscles are utilized.

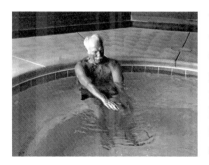

The right arm is extended with a flat palm in front of the torso on the water's surface. The left arm is moved to the left side. The palm is fisted. With a swinging motion, the left fisted palm is pulled under the straight right arm underneath the elbow. This movement is repeated 12 times.

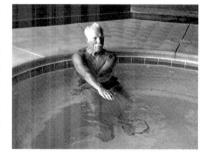

Fighting Arms

Both arms are placed at the sides of torso with bent elbows. The palms of the hands are in a fisted position. The right arm is pushed out two times as if punching something. Then the left fisted palm reaches across the torso, like a left hook in boxing. The left arm follows the same pattern, pushing out one or two times. The right fisted palms reaches across the torso, like a right hook in boxing. The arms and fisting movements are alternated for approximately 12 times.

The arms with bent elbows are placed near the sides of the torso. The palms are fisted.
See #1 below

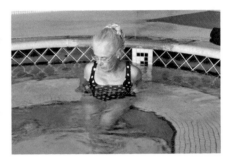

Photo 1: With the arms in this position near the sides of the torso, the Subscapularis and Latissimus dorsi are utilized.

The right arm with fisted palms is pushed out forward one or two times, as if punching. The left fisted palm reaches across the torso, like a left hook in boxing.

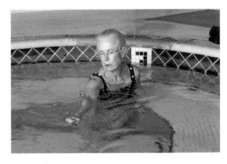

Photo 2: When the arm performs the punch, the anterior Deltoid, Serratus anterior, and Pectoralis major muscles are utilized. When the arm performs the swing, the anterior Deltoid, and Pectoralis major muscles are utilized.

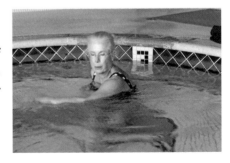

The left arm is pushed out forward, one or two times, as if punching. The right fisted arm reaches across the torso like a right hook in boxing. This movement is repeated for approximately 12 times.

23

Palm Scoops

Arms are floating on the water's surface, straight in front of the torso. Clasp both hands together by putting one thumb under the palm of the hand and bringing the second thumb over the top of the first thumb, like locking the thumbs together. Move the clasped hands to the left. Then, with hands still clasped, rotate the wrists and pull with the left arm downward toward the knees and up toward the right shoulder. The arms perform a "scooping" movement. Rotate the clasped hands and "scoop" toward the knees and the left shoulder. This "scooping" movement of the palms should be repeated for approximately 12 alternating times.

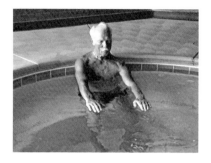 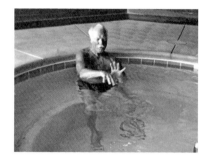 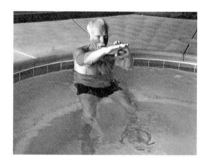

The arms are floating on the water's surface in front of the torso, palms are flat. Place the right thumb under the left palm; then put the left thumb over the right thumb, like "locking the thumbs."

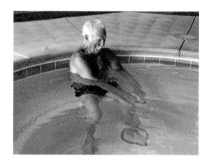 Rotate the right arm toward the knees and to the left shoulder. With a "scooping" movement of the left palm, pull the left arm downward and toward the right shoulder. Alternate "scooped" hands from left to right.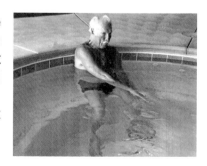

The following muscles and/or groups of muscles are utilized by performing this exercise: Pectoralis major, posterior Deltoids, middle Trapezius, Serratus anterior, lateral abdominals, and pelvic stabilizers.

"The Archer"

The torso is held in an upright position with a nice straight back for posture. This exercise can be done standing or sitting on a bench. Both arms are floating on the water's surface. The palms of both hands are brought together and pulled toward the left side of the torso staying just under the water's surface. The thumbs are kept up out of the water. The right palm is pulled across the left palm as if pulling a bow string. The thumb remains above the water's surface as the arm is drawn is across the torso and extended outward to the right side. The right arm is then brought in front of the torso with a circling movement in front of the torso, returning to the out-stretched left arm. This "archer" movement is repeated for 12 times with the right arm. Then, both arms are moved to the right side of the torso. The thumbs remain up; the arms are just below the water's surface. The thumb remains above the water's surface as the left palm is drawn back and across the torso toward the left side and extended outward. The left arm is then brought in front of the torso with a circling movement, returning to the out-stretched right arm. The "archer" movement is repeated 12 times with the left arm.

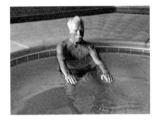 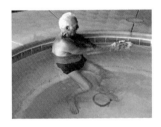 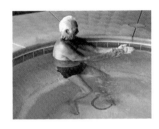 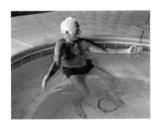

Both palms are held flat and together facing toward the left side, slightly below the water's surface. The thumbs are up. The right, flat palm is "drawn" across the left palm and in front of the torso until the right arm is fully extended outward. Then the right arm moves in a semi-circle with the thumb up out of the water, returning to the left palm. The "archer" is repeated 12 times.

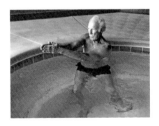 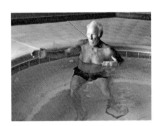 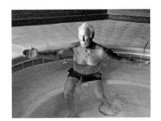 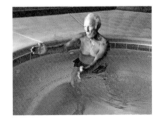

Both palms are held flat and together facing toward the right side of the torso, slightly below the water's surface. The thumbs are up. The left, flat palm is "drawn" across the right palm and in front of the torso until the left arm is fully extended outward. Then the left arm moves is a semi-circle with the thumb up out of the water, returning to the right palm. The "archer" movement is repeated 12 times.

"Drawing" of the arm across and in front of the torso is shoulder retraction. The posterior Deltoid, middle Trapezius, and the Triceps are utilized. **The "return"** and semi-circular motion of the arm is a horizontal shoulder adduction. The Triceps, anterior Deltoid and Pectoralis major are utilized.

Crossing Shoulder Stretch

Hands are placed upon the knees for this exercise.

The person is seated on the bench of the spa for this exercise. Knees are held in a slight V position with feet spread apart. The left hand is placed upon the right knee; the right arm is pushed across the torso on the surface of the water at an angle, like a reaching swim stroke. Then, the right hand is placed upon the left knee; the left arm is pushed across the torso on the surface of the water at an angle, like a reaching swim stroke. Repetition is alternately performed 12 times.

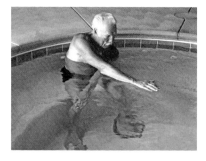

The person is seated on the bench, knees held in a slight V position with the feet spread apart. The left hand is place upon the right knee. The right arm is pushed across the torso on the surface of the water at an angle.

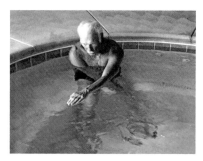

The seated position is the same as above. The right hand is placed upon the left knee. The left arm is pushed across the torso on the surface of the water at an angle.

This exercise challenges the Latissimus dorsi, Teres major, middle Trapezius, and Deltoid muscle groups. The "reaching action" is pulling the scapula around the torso engaging the Serratus anterior and the Pectoralis major. The elbow straightening is stretching the Triceps; the wrist extension is challenging the Extensors of the fingers and wrist. The pulling back of the arm challenges the middle Trapezius, posterior Deltoid and the Biceps. The alternating of the hand to the knee is an adduction at the shoulder of the anterior Deltoid and Pectoralis major. The "torso twist" of this exercise works the internal and external abdominal oblique muscles. The Erector spinae are stretched as are the Intercostal muscles and the middle Trapezius.

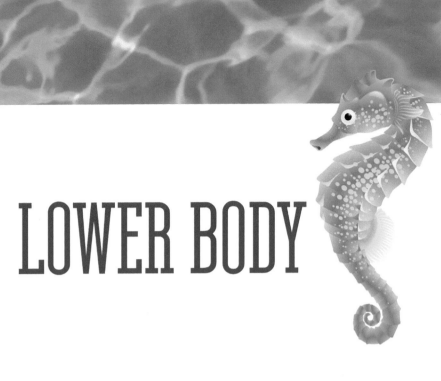

LOWER BODY

"At 75 years of age, I had a knee replacement. Water Therapy was what helped me get through the healing. After three years of therapeutic water exercises, I still benefit greatly."
– Joan N.

"With water therapy exercise, I am able to limber up and have more flexibility. I seldom have leg cramps like I used to have. I can sleep better and feel that I am truly a healthier person. I have a positive attitude and a healthier outlook on life." – Donna B.

"Having undergone extensive back surgery with multiple post-surgical complications, I am indebted to the therapeutic water exercises for "pulling through"– first, in strengthening my body sufficiently to suffer through the ordeal, and later in accelerating my full recovery." – Jane B.

Hip Hula

A bench is needed for this exercise.

Using the bench, chair, or stationary part of the Jacuzzi, rotate the hips in a circular motion. Lean the hips toward the right making a circular movement, shifting the shoulders above the hips for approximately 12 circles. Then, reverse and rotate the hips to the left for approximately 12 rotations.

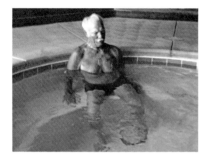

The person is seated comfortably on the bench with flat palms near the hips for support.

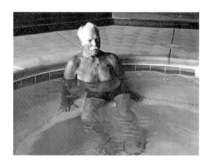

Lean the torso to the right, and lean slightly forward to circle and rotate the hips to the right. The upper torso makes a slight circle to the right to get and keep the hips rotating to the right.

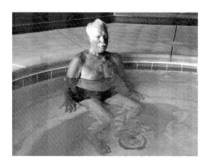

Lean the torso to the left, and lean slightly forward to circle and rotate the hips to the left. The upper torso makes a slight circle to the left to get and keep the hips rotating to the left.

This exercise encourages the stretching of the hip Abductors, hip Adductors, abdominals, and spinal Extensors are contracting.

Butterfly Knees

A bench is needed for this set of exercises.

To begin this exercise, the knees are held together; the palms are flat and placed upon the bench for support. The knees are then elevated slight above the bench. The feet are off the floor of the pool. The knees are moved in/out or back/forth like the wings of a butterfly. This "butterfly" movement of the knees is repeated for approximately 12 times.

The person is seated comfortably on the bench with flat palms near the hips for support. The knees are elevated slightly above the bench, which raises the feet off the pool floor.

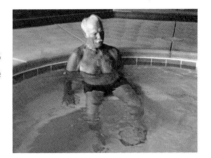

The knees are moved in/out or back and forth like the wings of a butterfly for approximately 12 times.

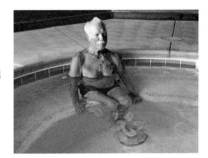

When this exercise is completed with the 12 times, the knees are left in an outward position.

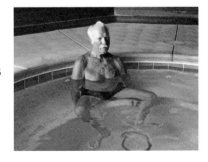

Keeping the knees together, moving them out and then drawing them back together requires contraction of the hip Adductors, principally the Adductor magnus, Pectineus and Gracilis muscles. Elevating the knees off the pool floor requires the hip Flexors, principally the Iliopsoas. To stabilize the torso the Extensors of the spine are contracting with the abdominal muscle. The exercising of the legs requires the Latissimus dorsi, abdominal muscles, and spinal Extensors. Paravertebral muscles are strengthened. Spreading the knees apart requires the hip Abductors, strengthening the Gluteus medius and Gluteus maximus muscles.

Hip Hike or "Swaying Hips"

This exercise is an alternating hip pull-up, designed to cause the lower back to sway from side to side. The knees are at a 90-degree angle. The soles of the feet are flat on the pool floor. Alternately the pull up of the heels, first the right and then the left. Leave the toes upon the pool floor. This gives the feeling of the hips rotating from side to side as if being pulled up.

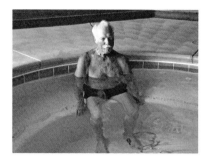

The soles of the feet are flat on the pool floor. The knees are at a 90-degree angle.

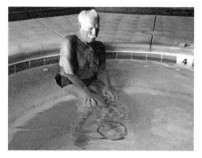

The torso leans slightly to the left. The right heel pulls upward, which cause the right hip to elevate. Alternate a right heel pull-up with a left heel pull-up.

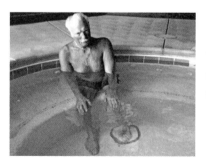

The torso leans slightly to the right. The left heel pulls upward, which causes the left hip to elevate. Alternate left heel pull-up with right heel pull-up.

The performance of this exercise utilizes the following muscles or muscle groups: Quadratus lumborum, lateral abdominals, spinal Extensors. The same muscle groups are utilized on both sides by alternating. When the right heel is pulled up, the ankle "performs" a plantar flexion movement. The pelvis lift of the hip challenges the Quadratus lumborum muscle.

Hip Walking (Optional)

A bench is needed for this exercise.

"Walk" the hips back and forth on the bench. Simply move the hips forward and backward on the bench. Movement forward and backward can be helped by leaning forward slightly at the shoulder and leading with bent elbows. The bent elbows near the hips will assist moving the torso forward and backward. Leading with the elbows by moving the shoulders will also help get the hips moving forward/backward. If the hips are actually pulled up and placed back down, this exercise is very beneficial to the lower spine and hip area. Note: This exercise can deteriorate a swim suit by scraping it on the bench. If the hips are actually pulled up and moved, the swim suit will not be scraped by the bench.

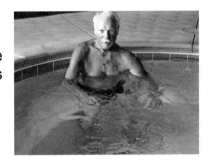

The hands are placed downward near the hips. The elbows are bent. The right bent elbow is moved forward as the hip elevates to "walk."

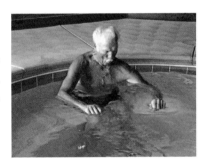

The lower torso moves forward at the hips. The hips propel the lower torso forward and backward. It appears to be more like a wiggle on the pool bench, but the hips do move. This exercise is felt in the lower spine.

If one places their hands upon the bench for support, the Latissimus dorsi are put into action. Without the hands upon the bench, the Quadratus lumborum are utilized.

Hip Pull-Ups

A bench is need for the following exercises.

The person is seated on a bench. The hands are placed next to the torso for support. Knees are slightly flexed; feet are flat on the pool floor. The hips are pulled up toward the front of the body. The palms of the hands help push the hips up, and the arms become straight. As the hips come down, the arms relax. This upward/downward movement is repeated about 12 times.

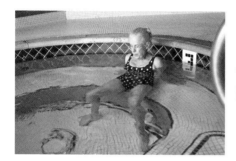

The person is seated at the bench; palms are flat on on the bench beside the torso and even with hips.

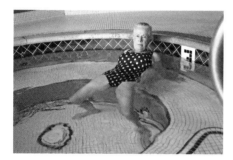

The hips are pulled up and the arms straighten as they push up the hips.

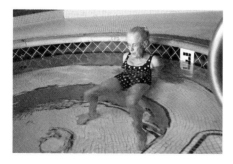

The arms relax and let the hips come back down to to the bench.

The movement/flexion of the hips is a concentric contraction of the Iliopsoas muscle. The shoulder depressions, as the hips are pulled up, aids in the pelvis elevation, and challenges the Latissimus dorsi, Gluteus maximus, and the Triceps muscles. When the arms relax and the muscles contract, the same muscles perform an eccentric muscle contraction.

Hip Pull-Up with Knee/Ankle Movement

This exercise extends the Hip Pull Ups of the previous exercise. To perform this exercise, keep the hips elevated with arms straight and heel supporting from the pool floor. The right ankle is pulled underneath and in back of the left knee; the left ankle is pulled under the right knee. This ankle movement is alternated between right and left ankle being placed under and in back of the opposite knee. The exercise is only repeated for 3 or 4 times for each ankle placement. **This exercise can be stressful on the shoulders if repeated for more than 3 or 4 times.**

The person elevates the hips by straightening the arms which remain on the bench near the hips.

Photo #1 (right): The movement is the same as the previous exercise. This movement is a concentric/eccentric contraction of the Triceps, the Latissimus dorsi and the Gluteus maximus.

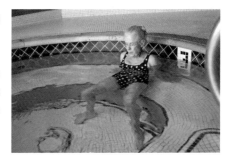

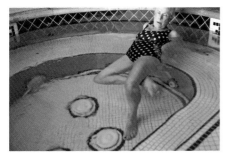

The right ankle is placed under the left knee; the left ankle is placed under the right knee. The ankle movement is alternated for **no more than** 3 or 4 times.

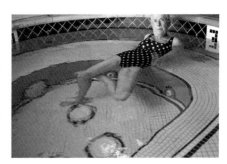

Photo #2 (above): The knee flexion to clear the opposite leg requires the Hamstring muscles to contract. The thigh rotation stretches the hip Flexors and hip Abductors.

33

Heel Taps and Leg Stretches

A bench is needed for the next series of exercises.

The person is seated on the pool bench. Flat palms are placed next to the torso on the bench if the person needs to brace himself/herself. The back is held straight for good posture. The knees are at a 90-degree angle to the pool floor; knees and ankles are together. This is simply performed by: right heel, right straight leg; left heel, left straight leg.

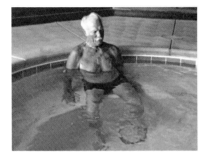

The person is seated on the pool bench. Flat palms are placed next to the torso on the bench to brace the torso. The knees are at a 90-degree angle to the pool floor; knees and ankles are together.

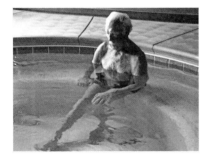

The right heel is extended and placed on the pool floor, toes pointing toward the surface of the water. Return the leg to the starting position. Then, the left heel is extended and placed on the pool floor, toes pointing toward the top of the water. Return the leg to the starting position. Repeat a total of 12 times.

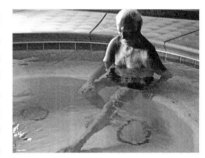

This toe point movement of the foot upward is a concentric/eccentric contraction of the Triceps, Latissimus dorsi and Gluteus maximus. Pointing the toes to the surface of the water requires ankle dorsiflexion by the anterior Tibialis muscles. It also stretches the Soleus muscle if the knee is flexed. The Gastrocnemius muscle is stretched when the knee is straight. Returning to the starting point in this exercise stretches many of the same muscles as the previous exercise. However, there is a sustained contraction of the anterior Tibialis muscle.

Toe Points

Legs are together at the knees and ankles at a 90-degree angle to the pool floor. To make this exercise easier to perform the feet may need to be slightly extended in front of the torso. Point toes toward the pool floor, moving the heels upward. (The water's buoyancy will help keep the legs up.) Then, point both toes toward the ceiling/sky moving the heels downward. If additional support is needed, put arms with flat palms near the sides of the torso. Point both toes to the pool floor; then, point both toes to the ceiling/sky 12 times.

The knees and ankles are at a 90-degree angle to the pool floor. Toes are pointed to the pool floor. Then, the toes are pointed to the ceiling/sky.

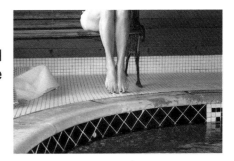

Pull up the toes so that both heels touch the pool floor. Alternate toes/heels for a total of 12 times. The exercise is designed to use both feet together.

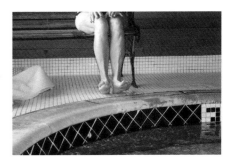

This particular part of the exercise works the Gastrocnemius and Soleus muscles.

Alternate Heel-Toe Points

The knees are at a 90-degree angle to the pool floor, and the ankles are fairly close together. Pull up the heels so the toes are pointing toward the bottom of the pool as in the previous exercise. Then, pull up the right toes so that the right heel and left toes are on the bottom of the pool. Point the toes and then, the heels on the bottom of the pool, moving only the ankles. Alternate toe/heel and heel/toe keeping the ankles fairly close together for 12 times. (Example: right heel/left toe and then right toe/left heel).

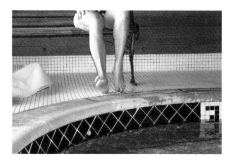

Knees are at a 90-degree angle to the pool floor. Ankles are together. Pull up the heels and point both toes toward the bottom of the pool. The toe and heel are then alternated toward the pool floor. Right heel is on the pool floor; left toe points to the pool floor.

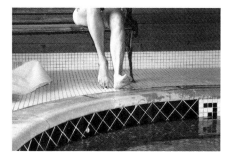

Simply change, left heel on pool floor; right toe points to the pool floor, and alternate the toe/heel and heel/toe until completion of 12 alternations.

The pulling up of the heels stretches the Peroneus longus, posterior Tibialis and the Soleus of the foot. Placing the heels upon the pool floor and pulling up the toes contracts the anterior Tibialis, the Extensor hallucis longus, and the Extensor digitorum longus.

Leg Lifts

Seated on the bench with knees at a 90-degree angle to the pool floor and with knees together, first pull up one foot, and then the other, alternating legs and lifting from the knees. Repeat this alternating movement of the legs for approximately 12 times total, which would give each leg a series of 6 times. When the alternating of the legs is complete, follow by lifting both legs together for another 12 times. If support is needed, the palms maybe placed beside the torso on the bench, arms straight.

Knees and ankles are together. The knees angle at 90-degrees to the pool floor as one is seated on the bench. The back remains as straight as possible. If support is needed, the hands are placed, with flat palms, on the bench.

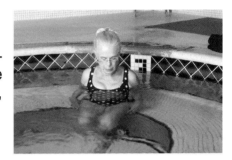

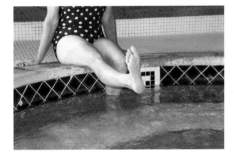

First, the right leg is lifted to make the leg straight. Then, the left leg is lifted to make the left leg straight. Alternate legs 6 times for each leg, making a total of 12 times for both legs.

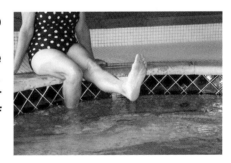

Quadriceps are strengthened when straightening the knee, and stretched when bending the knee.

Knees and ankles are together. The knees are at a 90-degree angle to the pool floor as one is seated on the bench. For added support, the arms, with flat palms are placed near the sides on the bench. Both legs are lifted at the same time to straighten the legs while keeping the back as straight as possible. It may be necessary to lean the torso slightly backwards against the pool wall. The object of this exercise is to straighten the legs from a seated position. This exercise should be repeated for 12 times.

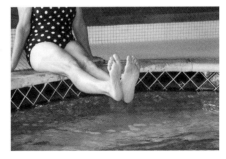

Note: Progressive implementations of this exercise would be non-use of the hands for support to allow core muscles to strengthen stability of the torso and strengthen abdominal muscles while exercising.

Calf Slides (Toes Up and Heel Down)

A bench is needed for this exercise.

With buttocks on the bench and hands near the torso for support if needed, place both legs straight in front of the torso. The toes point upward. Placing the right toe on the left ankle, slide the right toe up to the left knee. Rotate the ankle so toes point outward and slide the right heel back down the left calf to the ankle, the knee is slightly outward. Then change to the right leg using the left foot. Placing the left toe on the right ankle, slide the left toe up to the right knee. Rotate the ankle so toes point outward and slide the left heel back down the right calf to the ankle. The knee is slightly outward. The legs remain up toward the water's surface the entire exercise. Repeat 12 times.

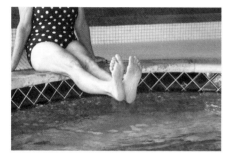

The hands are near the torso for support if needed. Both legs are placed straight in front of the torso. The toes point upward.

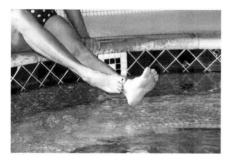

Placing the right toe on the left ankle, slide the right toe up the left calf to the left knee. Rotate the ankle so toes point outward and slide the right heel back down the left calf to the ankle.

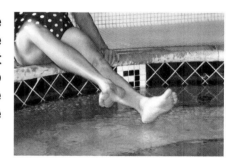

Then, placing the left toe on the right ankle, slide the left toe up to the right knee (not shown in above photos). Rotate the ankle so toes point outward and slide the left heel back down the right calf to the ankle.

The movement of placing the right toe upon the left ankle, and vice versa, dorsiflexes the foot, challenging the anterior Tibialis. The Sartorius and Iliopsoas are also working to do movement at the hip. The movement of sliding the heel down to the ankle activates the Quadriceps and the Gluteus maximus. The ankle remains dorsiflexed by the anterior Tibialis.

Knee Swings/Knee Wags

A bench is needed to perform this exercise.

The knees are bent and at a 90-degree angle to the bench. Knees and ankles are together and the feet are flat on the pool floor. The right, bent knee is moved out and back/out and in like the one wing of a butterfly. This movement is repeated for 12 times. Then, the left, bent knee is moved out and back/out and in like the one wing of a butterfly. This same movement is repeated for 12 times.

The knees are bent with ankles together and at a 90-degree angle. Toes may or may not be flexed and feet do not necessarily need to be flat.

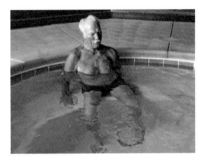

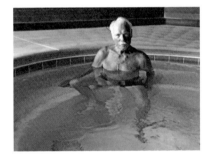 The right knee is moved out and back/out and in like the one wing of a butterfly for 12 times. This same movement is repeated with the left knee, out and back/out and in like the one wing of a butterfly for 12 times.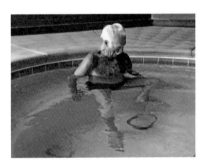

This exercise helps stabilize the back by working the Multifidus, Erector spinae and transverse abdominals. When the legs are moved outward the hip Abductors are strengthened and stretched. When the legs are moved inward the hip Abductors (Gluteus maximus; Gluteus medius; Gluteus minimus; Tensor fasciae) are strengthened and stretched. The pulling up of the knee is causing the Iliopsoas muscle to stay firmly fixed in one position. Moving the knee and leg outward and to the side stretches the hip Adductors.

"Grape Stomping"

Buttocks at the edge of bench.

The knees are bent and at a 90-degree angle to the pool floor. The person needs to sit erect throughout the exercise, supporting the torso with the hands on the bench if necessary. The feet are flat on the pool floor. Move the knees out to the side with the upper legs forming a large V shape. Pull up first the right knees/foot and then the left knees/foot, alternating the knees and feet, like stomping grapes. Use the heels to tap the pool floor after each repetition. Make sure the knees are coming up toward the water's surface, approximately 4-5 inches from the pool floor.

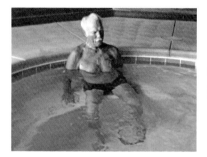

For the beginning position, the legs are bent at a 90-degree angle. Knees and ankles are together. The feet are flat on the pool floor.

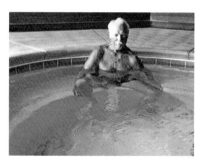

To start this exercise, the knees are moved apart to make a large V shape. The feet are flat on the pool floor.

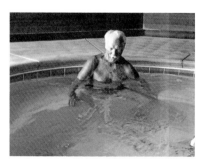

Each knee is pulled up, alternating right/left and tapping the pool floor with the flat foot or the heel of each foot. This stomping is repeated right/left with each heel/foot 12 times.

The Quadriceps muscles are stabilizing. The lifting motion activitates the Iliopsoas muscle. Pushing downward works the Gluteus maximus, Gluteus minimus and medius. The Adductor longus, Pectineus, and Gracilis muscles are also strengthened and stretched.

"Froggy"

Buttocks at the edge of bench.

Both knees are placed in a large V shape. The soles of the feet are brought up and clapped together, like clapping hands. The arms with flat palms are at the sides of the torso, supporting the body. The feet are placed back on the pool floor between foot claps.

To begin this exercise, the knees are apart in a large V shape. The soles of the feet are flat on the pool floor.

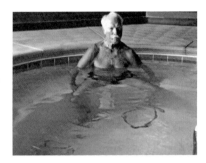

The torso is supported by straight arms with palms flat on the bench both legs are raised as the soles of the feet come together to clap/touch in front of the torso. This is like clapping of hands only the soles of the feet are clapping instead.

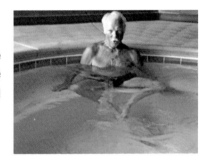

The knees are up and out, which strengthens and stretches the following muscles groups: Iliopsoas, Gluteus maximus, and lateral Hamstrings. When the knees are down and in the following muscle groups are strengthened and stretched: Gluteus maximus, Adductor longus, Adductor magnus, Gracilis, and Pectineus. Ankle is placed in an inversion/eversion position. The inversion activates the posterior Tibialis. The torso being stabilized throughout this exercise enables the Latissimus dorsi, abdominal muscles, spinal Extensors, and the paravertebral muscles to be strengthened. Hips are performing an external rotation stretching and strengthening the Iliopsoas, Adductor longus, Brachialis, Pectineus muscles. The flexion of the hips works the Rectus femoris, and Iliopsoas. The adduction of the hips stretches the Gluteus medius and Gluteus maximus.

"Froggy" Extend

Buttocks at the edge of bench.

As you sit on the bench, the knees are kept apart in a big V shape. Straight arms with flat palms are beside the torso for support. The soles of the feet are pulled up and clapped together. Then clapped feet are brought up and extended out in front of the torso. With the soles of the feet remaining together, the feet are pushed and pulled back and forth. The knees bend to the side with each push/pull. This exercise should be repeated 12 times.

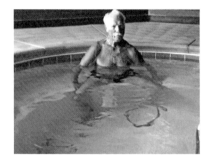

To begin this exercise, the bent knees are moved to the side at a 60-degree angle to make the shape of a big V. The arms are held at the sides of the torso, palms flat on the bench, to support the torso.

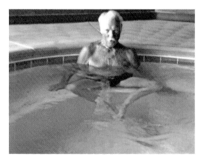

The soles of the feet are brought up together as if clapping hands, but with the soles of the feet.

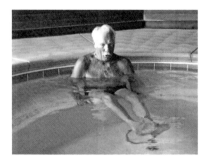

The "clapped" feet are pushed and pulled back and forth. The knees go out to the side. This push/pull movement should be repeated for approximately 12 times.

Abductor muscles are strengthened and stretched. Iliopsoas, Adductor longus, and Gluteus maximus muscle groups are strengthened and stretched.

"Ankle Flexies" Plus

The knees are bent at a 90-degree angle as if seated in a chair, and the feet are on the pool floor. Pull up the right, lower leg and "wave" to the bottom of the pool, which flexes the ankles. "Wave" the foot, flexing the ankle, to the bottom of the pool about 12 times. Keeping the lower leg elevated, rotate the ankle inward; then rotate the ankle outward for a total of 12 circles.

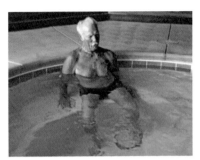

Knees and ankles are at a 90-degree angle to the bench as if seated in a chair. The feet are flat on the pool floor.

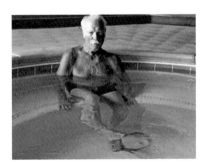

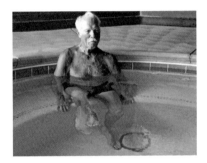 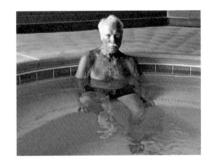

The right lower leg is pulled up slightly from the pool floor. The foot is flexed, like waving to the pool floor, foot "waves" down and up, for 12 ankle flexes. Then, the same right ankle is moved inward and "circled" inward (counter clockwise) 12 times. Following the inward ankle rotation, the ankle is then "circled" outward (clockwise) for 12 times. This same movement is repeated for the left ankle so that each ankle is flexed and rotated both inward and outward.

In this exercise, when the foot is pulled up, the Iliopsoas is challenged to hold the leg up from the pool floor. The upward movement of the foot activates the anterior Tibialis, stretches the Soleus and posterior Tibialis. The downward movement stretches the anterior Tibialis.

Calf Stretch

The buttocks are at edge of the bench.

The legs are extended out in front of the torso. The water buoyancy will help hold up the legs. The hands with flat palms are out to the side of the torso to support the torso. The knees and ankles are together. Point the toes upward (original position); then, flex the toes, point them away from the forehead and hold in that position for about 30 seconds. This is not an easy exercise.

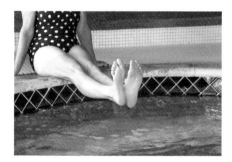

Straight legs are extended out in front of the torso. The water buoyancy will help hold up the legs. The hands with flat palms are out to the side of the torso to support the torso. The knees and ankles are together. The soles of the feet are flat. Point the toes upward (original position).

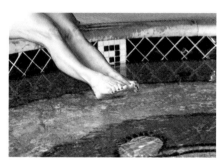

Then flex the toes, and point them away from the forehead and hold in that position for about 30 seconds.

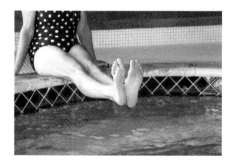

The toes are then pointed upward and towards the forehead (flexed a little further back than the original position) after being held for 30 seconds. The point/flex of the toes is repeated for as many times as possible working up to 12 times.

With this exercise, the abdominals are stabilizing. The hip Adductors, ankle dorsiflexors, Iliopsoas, anterior Tibialis, and the Extensor digitorum longus and brevis are all being stretched and strengthened.

Ankle Rotation

Knees and ankles are together and legs are at a 90-degree angle. Using only the right foot, pull up the toe, put the toe back down, the heel comes slightly upward. The right foot rolls along the outside of the foot from toes to heel. The toe is pulled up just long enough to roll the right foot back and place the whole foot down on the pool floor to its original position. The rotation/roll of the right foot is repeated 12 times. The same exercise is performed with the left foot. The left foot toe is elevated and placed back down; the heel comes slightly upward. The outside of the left foot rolls to the heel, pull the toe up just long enough to roll the left foot to the toe and place it back down on the pool floor. The left foot "rolls" for 12 times.

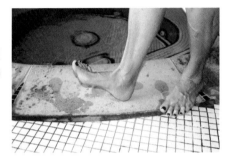

The knees are at a 90-degree angle to the pool floor, and ankles are together. (Photo of beginning position not shown.) The right foot toe is pulled upward.

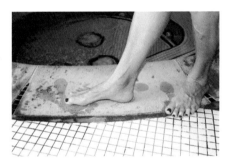

The right foot toe is placed back down on the pool floor. The heel comes up slightly.

This movement is a plantar flexion by the Soleus muscle.

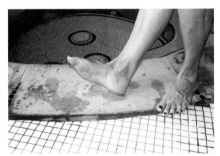

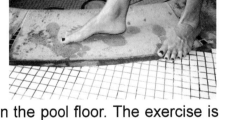

(Photo at left) The right foot is then rolled along the outside of the foot from toe to heel. The toe is pulled up just long enough to roll the right foot back to its original position.
(Photo at right) The foot once again becomes flat upon the pool floor. The exercise is repeated for 12 times. Then, this same exercise is performed with the left foot.

Rolling out is a concentric movement by the posterior Tibialis muscle as an ally to the movement. The rolling inward stretches the Peroneus longus muscle.

45

Heel Taps and Foot Rolls

The knees are at a 90-degree angle to the pool floor with ankles together. Stretch the right leg out in front of the torso as far as possible so it is straight with the heel resting upon the pool floor. Then, roll or tap the toe on the pool floor. Return the leg to its original 90-degree angle position after each heel tap/toe roll. Repeat the heel tap/toe roll 12 times. Then repeat the same exercise with the left leg making sure to return the leg to the 90-degree angle position   Repeat the toe taps to the left side 12 times as well.

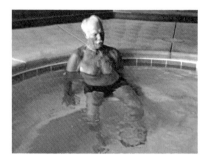

The knees and ankles are together as close as possible. The knees are at a 90-degree angle to the pool floor.

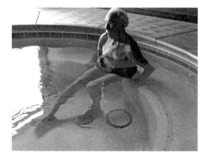

Extend the right leg out in front of the torso as far as possible making the leg become straight. Tap the heel and roll the toe to the pool floor for about 10 seconds. Repeat the heel taps/toe roll 12 times.

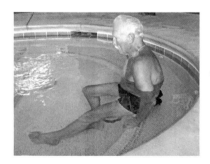

Repeat this same exercise for the left leg with the same 12 heel taps/toe rolls, and returning the foot leg to its original 90-degree angle position to the pool floor.

The movement of the leg is a hip abduction. The knee in the extension position is an alteration between ankle dorsiflexion and plantar flexion. The knee extension utilizes the Quadriceps; the ankle dorsiflexion utilizes the anterior Tibialis; the plantar flexion works the posterior Tibialis and Gastrocnemeus. The Latissimus dorsi is the principal stabilizer of the torso and shoulder depressor. Extending the knee requires the combined contraction of the Gluteus maximus and Quadriceps muscle groups. Rolling the foot into a downward pointed position requires contraction of the plantar Flexors of the ankle, principally the Gastrocnemius muscle, and stretches the anterior Tibialis muscle. Returning to the starting position requires the contraction of the hip Flexors, principally the Iliopsoas, Hamstring, and anterior Tibialis muscles.

Knee "Taps" with Heels

The knees and ankles remain at a 90-degree angle to the pool floor. The knees are separated enough to make a V shape with the knees. Pull the right heel up to tap the left knee and put it back down on the pool floor. Then the left heel is tapped to the right knee and put back down on the pool floor. This same movement is alternately repeated, right/left, for 12 knee taps.

The knees and ankles remain at a 90-degree angle to the pool floor. The knees are separated slightly enough to make a V shape with the knees.

The heel to the knee is a concentric movement, working the Ilioposoas, Hamstrings and Sartorius muscles.

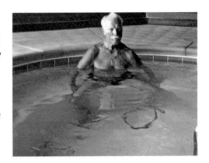

The right heel is pulled up from the pool floor into a position whereby it "taps" the left knee. The right heel returns to the pool floor after tapping the left knee. This knee tapping is repeated 12 times.

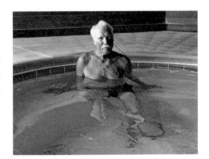

The left heel is pulled up to a position whereby it "taps" the right knee. The left heel returns to the pool floor after tapping the right knee. Repeat 12 times.

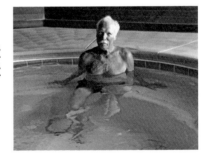

The heel movement to the knee is concentric. This movement causes the following muscles to "act": Iliopsoas, Sartorius and the Hamstrings. This exercise helps hip flexion and internal/external hip rotation. The Iliopsoas muscles in conjunction with the Sartorius muscles are stretched as the Gluteus maximus, Sartorius, and Quadriceps muscles straighten/lower the leg. The foot/ankle to opposite knee causes an external rotation of the thigh/hip activating the Sartorius. The knee flexion requires contraction of the Hamstrings.

Knee Touches with Knee

The knees remain at a 90-degree angle with the ankles together, feet on the pool floor. The knees are then moved and separated slightly with the upper legs forming a V shape, knees pointing outward. Tighten the tummy as if trying to blow up a balloon that will not expand. Pull up the right foot at the ankle to move the foot off the pool floor. Move the right knee to touch the left knee cap. Return right foot to floor. Then, pull up the left foot at the ankle enough to make the foot move off the pool floor. Move the left knee to tap the right knee cap. Alternate right and then left knee for 12 times.

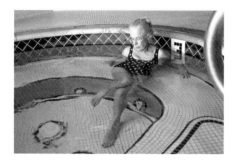

The right ankle is the pulled into a position whereby right knee moves and touches the left knee cap.

Photo #1: This part of the exercise involves a rotation of the thigh inward, a concentric contraction of the hip Adductors, and the Adductor magnus and longus.

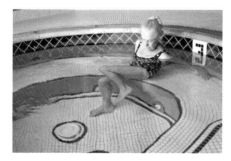

The left ankle is pulled up into a position whereby the left knee moves and touches the right knee.

Photo #2: This exercise rotates the thigh inward, a concentric contraction, activating the hip Adductors: Adductor magnus and longus. The hip extension activates the Gluteus maximus causing the Iliopsoas to stretch.

Knees to Armpits, Alternating

The person maintains a seated, erect posture position on the bench. Bent elbows help the arms to float on the water's surface a 90-degree angle. Alternating right/left, the knee is brought up to the armpit. This alternating movement of knee to armpit should be repeated for 12 times.

The person is seated on the bench. The arms are floating on the water's surface. The elbows are bent at a 90-degree angle and held even with the shoulders.

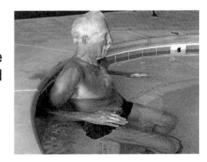

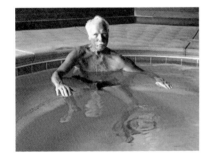

Alternating right/left, the knee is brought up as close as possible to the armpit.

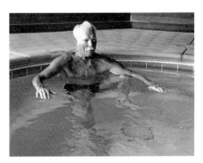

Maintaining an erect posture position on the bench without movement of the torso or pelvis requires a combined action of the muscles of the abdomen and spine, specifically the transverse abdominus and Multifidus muscle groups. The alternating movement of the hip when raising the knee to the armpit is stretching the hip Extensors, principally the Gluteus maximus muscles. Sitting and maintaining the opposite foot upon the pool floor is activating the hip Extensors, principally the Gluteus maximus in an isometric contraction.

Double Knee Lift

The person is seated on the bench. Flat palms are placed upon the bench for bracing the torso. The back is held straight for good posture. The knees and ankles are together and at a 90-degree angle to the pool floor. Both knees are pulled upward toward the chest at the same time and then placed back on the pool floor. This double pull of the knees should be repeated for 6 to 12 times.

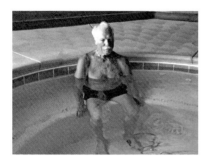

The person is seated on the bench. Flat palms are placed upon the bench for bracing the torso. The back is held straight for good posturing. The knees and ankles are at a 90-degree angle to the pool floor.

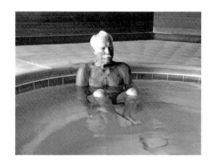

Both knees are pulled upward toward the chest at the same time and then placed back upon the pool floor.

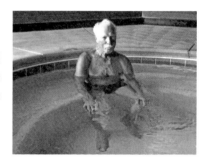

The Latissimus dorsi is the principal stabilizer of the torso and shoulder depressor. The hip Flexors bring the knees toward the chest. The hip Adductors maintain the proximity of the legs to each other while flexing the hips.

HANDS and WRISTS

The legs are bicycling like a stationary bike the entire time, and the fingers are moving throughout all of the following exercises.

Finger "Fans" (Palms Down)

The hands are comfortably held out in front of the torso, prone or flat to the surface of the water with the palms held down on the water's surface. The fingers, on both hands, are spread out as far as possible to the sides make the shape of a fan and the fingers on each hand are moved together keeping palms flat. The "fan" motion (spreading the fingers and moving them back together) is repeated for 12 to 25 times.

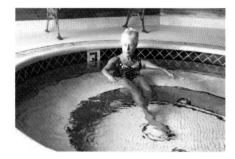

The palms are held down and flat, on the surface of the water. The fingers are together. Spread the fingers outward, making a fan shape, and then bring them back together. Repeat this "fan" shape for 12 to 25 times.

The fingers are spread apart and brought back together by a combination action of the palmar and dorsal Interossei muscles. The forearm position, supinated or pronated, gives a sense of muscle tension and effort. When the wrist is pronated, the tension is felt close to the elbow. When supinated, the tension is felt closer to the wrist. Author's opinion: The prone/pronated fans are assisted with stabilization by the pronators of the wrist on the palmar surface of the forearm. Supinated fans are assisted with stabilization of the Supinators of the wrist on the dorsum surface of the forearm.

Finger Fists (Palms Down)

The hands have just completed the fan motion from the previous exercise. The fingers are together in front of the torso. The palms remain down and flat, or prone, to the surface of the water. The fingers of both hands are then "fisted" and released. After releasing the fists while thrusting the fingers forward, the palms are again fisted. This fisting and releasing action of the fingers is repeated for 12 to 25 times.

The fingers are held together and the palms down and flat, or prone to the surface of the water in front of the torso. The fingers of both hands make a fist and release while thrusting the fingers forward and then fisting them again. This fist and release is repeated for 12 to 25 times.

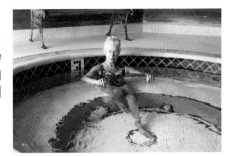

The flexion of the fingers challenges the Flexor digitorum longus and the Flexor digitorum profundus. The extension of the fingers challenges the Extensor digitorum communis.

Finger "Fans" (Palms Up)

The fingers on each hand are held together and the palms are held facing upward. The palms of the hands are floating on the water's surface. The fingers of both hands are spread out like fans and return to their original position. This "fan" shape with the palms up is repeated 12 to 25 times.

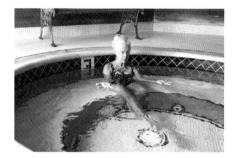

The fingers are held together, the flat palms are upward. The fingers of both hands spread out to the sides, like a fan, and return to their original position. This "fanning" action is repeated for 12 to 25 times.

When the fingers are held together with palms down, feasibly, the Flexor digitorum sublimus and Flexor digitorum profundus are stretched are spread widely; the open fingers engage the Extensor digitorum communis.

Finger Fists (Palms Up)

The fingers of both hands have just completed the fan motion with palms up. The fingers are together. The palms remain up and floating on the water's surface in front of the torso. The fingers of both hands are "fisted" and released with a forward thrust and then returned to a fisted position. This fisting and releasing action of the fingers with the palms up is repeated for 12 to 25 times.

The fingers are held together. The flat palms are held upward, floating on the water's surface. The fingers of both hands are "fisted" and thrust open. The fingers are then returned to a fisted position. The fisting and releasing action of the fingers is repeated 12 to 25 times.

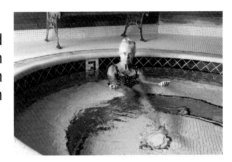

This exercise is a repeated version of the previous exercise so the same muscles are "engaged" and stretched during the exercise.

Piano

The palms of the hands are held downward, flat or prone to the water's surface. The fingers are extended, and slightly separated. Pull each finger down separately, both hands at the same time. This movement is like playing a piano with straight fingers. Repeat the finger movement starting with the thumbs and moving to the pinkie and back again to the thumbs. Repeat this movement for approximately 12 times.

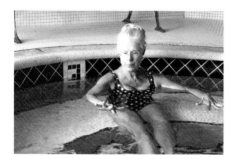

Holding the palms down and hands flat or prone to the surface of the water, with fingers extended and slightly separated. Pull each finger down separately, both hands at the same time. Begin the "piano" playing moving from the thumbs to the pinkie and back. Repeat this movement of "piano" playing for approximately 12 times.

This exercise "works" the fingers by flexing and extending them. When the fingers are flexed or bent, the Flexor digitorium profundus and sublimes are contracting. As the fingers are extended or straightened, the Extensor digitorum communis is contracting.

Claw Like A Cat

The hands are held in a relaxed position slightly below the water's surface. The fingers are moved like a clawing motion to the first knuckles. Then, the fingers become relaxed again. So this movement is like a claw/relax type of movement to the first knuckle of the fingers. The "clawing" movement is repeated for 12 times.

Both hands are held in front of the torso in a relaxed position slightly below the water's surface. The fingers are moved in a clawing motion to the first knuckles. Then, the fingers become relaxed again. The "clawing" movement is repeated for 12 times.

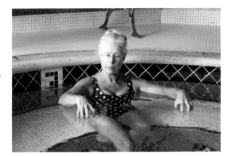

"Clawing" is principally a contraction of the Flexor digitorum profundus.

Thumb Circles (The Thumb Does Not Bend)

To begin this exercise, the person is seated on the bench of the pool. The hands are in front of the torso, and the palms are floating on the water's surface. The fingers of the hands are held comfortably. The thumbs of both hands inscribe a small circle toward the chest. The circling of the thumbs is performed for 12 to 25 times. Then the thumbs are reversed and are circled away from the seated person for the same number of thumb rotations, 12 to 25 times.

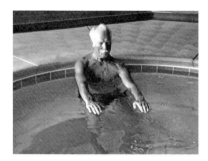

The person is seated on the bench. The hands are comfortably place in front of the seated person, held prone or flat to the water's surface with the palms down.

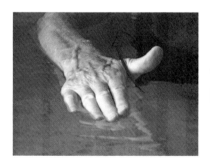

The thumbs on both hands are rotated toward the seated person for 12 to 25 thumb rotations.

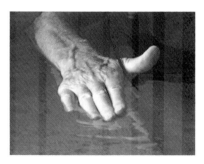

The hands are held flat on the water's surface with the palms down. **The thumbs of both hands are rotated away** from the seated person for 12 to 25 thumb rotations.

In sequence of the muscles being used, the circling motion of the thumbs stretches and contracts the Flexor pollicis longus, the Abductor pollicis, the Extensor pollicis, and the Adductor pollicis.

Thumb Stretches

The person is seated on the bench of the pool. The hands and arms are placed in front of the torso, and the flat palms are floating the water's surface. The fingers of the hands are held comfortably. The thumbs on both hands are pulled under the palms of the hands and brought back out again. This thumb stretching movement is repeated for 12 to 25 times.

The person is seated on the bench of the pool. The arms and hands are placed in front of the torso, and the flat palms are floating on the water's surface. The thumbs on both hands are pulled under the palms of the hands and brought back out again.

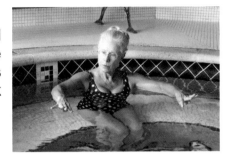

As the thumb comes outward, the Extensor pollicis is utilized; the inward thumb movements inward utilize the Opponens pollicis.

Wrist Circles

The person is seated comfortably on the pool bench. The arms and hands are in front of the torso. The palms of the hands are held flat or prone on the water's surface. The elbows are slightly bent. The wrist of both hands are circled inward for 12 to 25 times and then circled outward for 12 to 25 times.

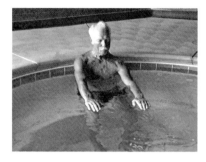

The person is seated comfortably on the pool bench. The arms and hands are held in front of the torso with the palms down.

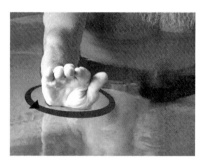

The elbows are slightly bent as both wrists circle at the same time, first, #1, **inward...**

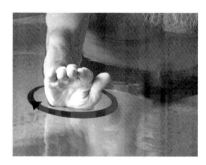

...and then, second, #2, **outward**.

In sequence, the following muscles are challenged: Extensor carpi, radials longus and brevus, Flexor carpi, Radialis, Ulnaris, and Flexor carpi.

UPPER BODY STRETCHES

"I had surgery 6 months ago. Water therapy classes have helped my range of motion and increased my strength. They are gentle on my body." – Ginny W.

"I experienced an injury to my right upper arm which halted my good times on the tennis courts. My doctor suggested a chiropractor. I worked with him for some time and then chose water therapy. The chiropractor released me in short time. The water therapy sessions were a great part of my healing." – Gretchen T.

"I have had two right shoulder surgeries, which failed, a right hip replacement, and a lower back fusion. I have experienced many courses of physical therapy. I have found that water therapy the most helpful of all. I have increased my balance and coordination." – Dr. Sheila F.

"Knee Hammer"

The person is seated on the bench with knees and ankles making a slight V. The left arm remains comfortable while the right arm is stretched outward and straight, palm into a fist. The fist is pulled downward to touch the right knee. The right fist is then pulled up and down from the knee position about 3 to 4 inches. Keep the fist below the waist. Perform this up and down movement with the right fist for 12 times. Then the right fist is moved left to right in front of the knees. Repeat with the left straight arm and fisted hand for 12 times.

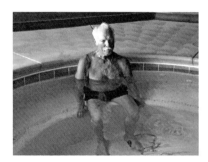

Photo 1: The knees and ankles are at a 90-degree angle to the pool floor. The knees are moved into a slight V shape.

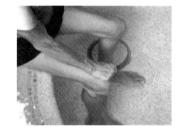
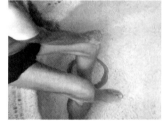

Photo 2 (at left): The right straight arm is stretched outward. The hand is clenched into a fist. The right fist is brought down to the right knee.
Photo 3 (at right): The fist is pulled up and down from the knee position about 3 to 4 inches. Tap knee 12 times. Keeping the fist in front of the knees move it side to side (right to left). Repeat 12 times.

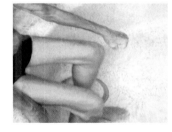
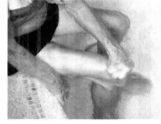

Photo 4 (at left): The left arm is stretched outward. The palm is clenched into a fist. The left fist is pulled down to the left knee.
Photo 5 (at right): The fist is moved up and down about 3 to 4 inches. Tap knee 12 times. Keeping the fist in front of the knees move it side to side (left to right). Repeat 12 times.

The downward movement is a series of concentric contractions which involves the following muscle and/or muscle groups: Latissimsu dorsi, anterior Deltoid, Pectoralis, and Teres major. The upward move involves concentric contractions of the Supraspinates, upper Trapezius, and Deltoid muscles.

The forward movement toward the midline of the torso requires the use of the Pectorialis and the anterior Deltoid muscles. The movement away from the midline of the torso requires the use of the posterior Deltoid and middle Trapezius muscles.

Elbows Pull/Shoulder Stretch

The elbows are at a 90-degree angle, floating on the water surface, and slightly forward from the chest. Palms are flat, facing down to the pool floor. Both elbows are pulled back simultaneously to become even and in line with the shoulders. The elbows can be pulled backward beyond the chest with caution for an even greater shoulder stretch. This pull should be done 12 times. As a person masters the pull, the elbows can be brought further back from the chest, but not to exceed 2 inches.

The elbows are at a 90-degree angle, slightly forward from the chest. The arms are floating on the water's surface.

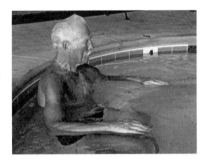

The elbows are pulled back at the same time to become in line with the shoulders and beyond the chest. This pull should be repeated 12 times.

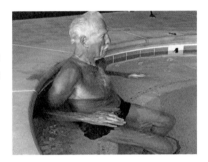

The stretch of this exercise requires the use of the Pectoralis major. This exercise also strengthens the middle Trapezius and posterior Deltoid.

Clam Scoop/Arm Stretches

The arms are extended in front of the torso near the surface of the water. The fingers are spread apart and brought together in front of the torso making a large circle. The fingers, remaining spread apart, are "scooped" into the chest. The palms are then reversed and with a pushing motion, the fingers are moved away from the chest as the arms straighten. This scooping/pushing motion is repeated for 12 times.

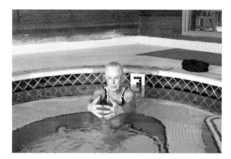

Photo 1: The arms are extended in front of the torso near the surface of the water. The fingers are spread apart and brought together in front of the torso making a large circle, like a balloon.

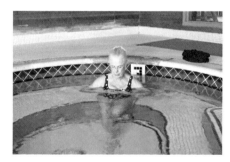

Photo 2: The fingers remain spread apart and are "scooped" into the chest.

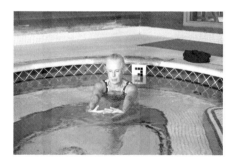

Photo 3: The palms are then reversed with a pushing motion, the fingers are pushed away from the chest as the arms straighten. This scooping/pushing motion is repeated 12 times.

Photos #1 and #2: The middle and posterior Deltoid as well as the Biceps are utilized at this step of the exercise.

Photo #3: This part of the exercise requires the use of the Pectoralis major and Tricep muscle groups.

Side Stretch/Reach for the Ankles

The person is seated on the bench with knees at a 90-degree angle. The right arm slides down the right calf of the leg as close to the ankle as possible. Return to starting position. Then, the left arm slides down the left calf of the leg as far down the calf and reaching down as close to the ankle as possible. This "slide" down the calf is repeated for each calf 6 times making a total of 12 times.

The person is seated on the bench. The right hand, flat palm, is extended and slides down the right calf reaching as close to the ankle as possible.

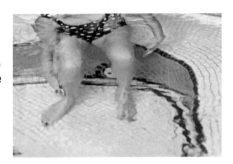

The left hand, flat palm, is extended and slides down the left calf of the leg reaching as close to the ankle as possible.

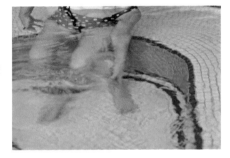

To reach, slide and stretch to touch the near the ankle is a flexion of the torso challenging the "six pack"/Rectus abdominus. The extension of the torso on the opposite side challenges the Erector spinae.

Arm Pull/Back Stretch

The right thumb or fist is placed underneath the left arm, and the thumb/fist reaches up to hook the arm above the elbow. Then, the right arm pulls the bent left arm across the torso. The left arm floats on the water's surface. The right thumb is dropped and the left thumb/fist is placed underneath the right arm, and the thumb/fist reaches up to hook the bent arm from behind. The right thumb pulls the bent right arm across the torso. The right arm floats on the water's surface. The motion of this exercise is kept fluid as the thumb is dropped and changed from side to side, alternating left/right arms. This fluid exchange of motion needs to be repeated 12 times.

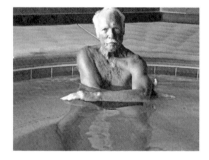 The right thumb or fist is placed underneath the left arm, and the thumb/fist reaches up to hook the bent arm from behind. The right arm pulls the bent left arm across the torso. Then, the thumb or fist is dropped.

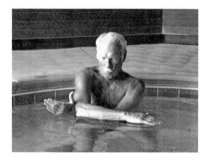 The left thumb/fist is placed underneath the right arm, and the thumb/fist reaches up to hook the bent arm from behind. The left arm pulls the bent right arm across the torso. Then, the thumb/fist is dropped. The exercise is repeated 12 times.

This part of the exercise stretches the posterior Deltoid, middle Trapezius, and Triceps muscles.

NECK

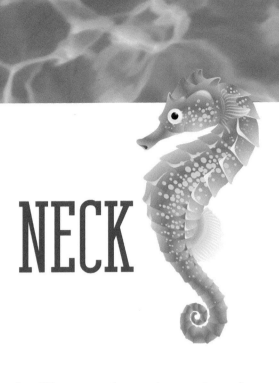

"The water therapy has made such an improvement in my neck. I had given up hope of regaining movement after neck surgery."
– Leila K.

"Recovery from a sprained ankle and 2 surgeries, 1 on my neck, were made easier with the water therapy classes, and the friendships which I made in the classes I took" – Claire A.

"Water therapy classes have helped me recover better from my knee replacement. I 'love' how it has helped all my joints."
– Debbie K.

Modeling?

The arms are bent at the elbow, a 90-degree position, and remain there. The right elbow is drawn back and the person looks over the left shoulder. The elbow is brought back, and the person looks straight ahead. Then, the left elbow is drawn back and the person looks over their right shoulder. This "modeling" and drawing back of the elbow, looking over the opposite shoulder, is repeated for 6 times.

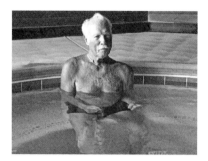

The elbows are bent at a 90-degree angle and held at the waist.

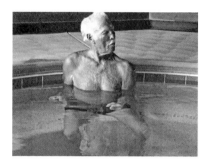

The person draws the right elbow back and looks over the left shoulder. Then the head is brought to the original position, looking straight ahead.

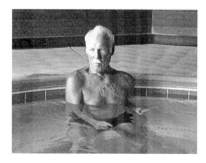

The elbows remain bent at a 90-degree angle and held at the waist. The person draws the left elbow back and looks over the right shoulder. Then, the head and elbows are brought back to their original position, straight forward.

The rotation of the torso requires the use of the following muscles: internal and external abdominals, obliques, and opposite Erector spinae. The stretch requires the use of the following muscles: Sternocleidomastoid, Scaleni, cervical thorasic and the Erector spinae, working the muscles on the side opposite to the direction in which the body is turning.

"Freeway" Exercise/Looking Back

Hands are placed upon the knees for this exercise.

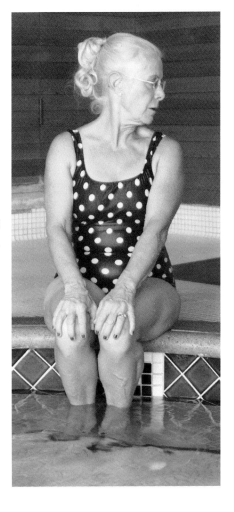

The head is turned slowly first to the right and then slowly to the left, while holding the head level as if looking forward. This "looking" is repeated 3 times.

Stretching of the Sternocleidomastoid muscles takes place with this exercise. Cervical Extensors are put into use on opposite sides.

Pendulum Neck Stretch

Hands are placed upon the knees for this exercise.

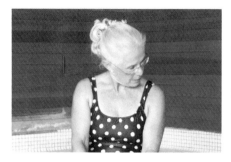

The head is turned **slowly** to look at the left shoulder, the head is kept upward and above the shoulder. Then, the chin is lowered toward the left shoulder and **slowly** moved to the right shoulder.

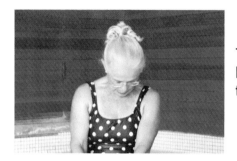

The chin moves and traces a slight curve across the collar bones. The head is brought slightly upward looking toward the right and above the shoulder.

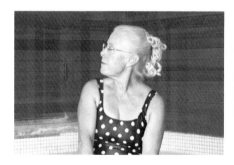

The chin is brought **slowly** down toward the chest and **slowly** back to the left shoulder, making the same curve in the opposite direction. Complete 3 to 4 times, making left to right and back 1 repetition.

This exercise stretches the Splenius capitus, and Erectus capitus.

Nods

Hands are placed upon the knees for this exercise.

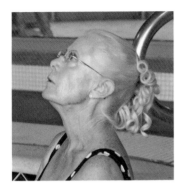

The person starts by looking straight ahead. The chin is "nodded" up and down from the chest to the straight position.

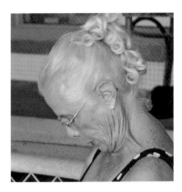

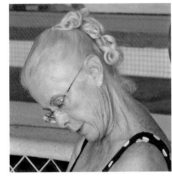

After the third repetition, the chin remains on the chest and is turned **no more than** 1 inch first to the left and then the right.

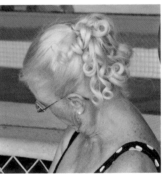

The YES/NO's of this exercise stretch the Erectus capitus and Splenius capitus

Turtle Pull

Hands are placed upon the knees for this exercise.

The person is looking straight ahead. The arms are pulled back parallel to the torso. The hands are placed at mid-thigh position or behind the buttocks, so that the shoulders feel as if the hands are in the back pocket of a pair of jeans.

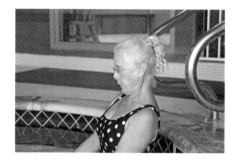

The chin is pulled inward toward the spine, and then pushed outward to the original position.

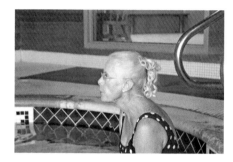

After the third repetition, the chin remains pulled back to the spine and is turned **no more than** 1 inch from left to right.

This exercise is a challenge to the neck Extensors and cranial Extensors.

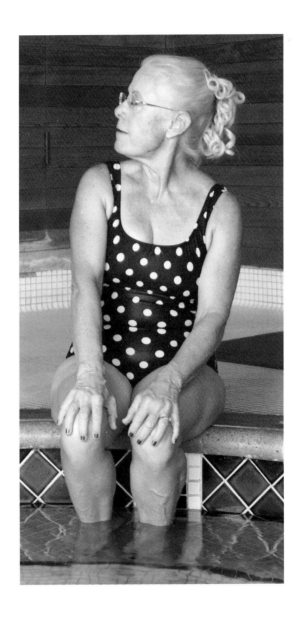

Esther Williams Swimwear (1983) compliments of Coral and Jade Apparel

www.coralandjadeapparel.com

References

American Exercise Association. *Aquatic Fitness Professional Manual.* Life Art Collections. Tech Pool Studios. Cleveland. Ohio. 1995.

Arthritis Foundation. *Arthritis foundation YMCA aquatic program.* Arthritis Foundation. Atlanta. Georgia. 1990.

Denomme, L. *Integrated Core Training.* ATRI National Aquatic Specialty Certificate Conference. Las Vegas. Nevada. 2010.

Dunkin, Mary Anne, Rath, Linda, Melone, Linda, Vargo, Bryan D. *Arthritis Today,* Arthritis Foundation. Vol. 26 No. 3. May-June 2012.

Gray, Henry, F.R.S. *ANATOMY Descriptive and Surgical.* Running Press. Philadelphia, Pennsylvania.1974.

Haggerty, M, Mitchell, T, and Sova, R. *ATRI hip and back specialty certificate manual.* ATRI. West Palm Beach. Florida. 2010.

Klapper, R.M.D., and Huey, L. *Heal Your Knees: How to Prevent Knee Surgery & What to Do If You Need It.* M. Evans and Company Inc. Lanham. New York. Boulder. Toronto. Plymouth. United Kingdom. 2004.

Klapper, R.M.D., and Huey, L. *Heal Your Hips: How to Prevent Hip Surgery and What to Do If You Need It.* John Wiley & Sons, Inc. New York. Chichester. Weinhem. Brisbane. Singapore. Toronto. 1999.

Kendall, F.P.PT, and McCreary, E.K., B.A. *MUSCLES Testing and Function* Williams & Wilkins. Baltimore. London. 1983.

Konno, J. *Ai Chi-flowing aquatic energy.* Port Washington DSL. 1996.

Hirschi, G. *MUDRAS--- yoga in your hands.* Samuel Weiser. York Beach. Maine. 2000.

Seiger, Lon H. and Hesson, James. *Walking for Fitness.* Brown & Benchmark. Dubuque. Iowa. 1994.
   Abstract: This book was listed as a reference because "approximately 87% of all Americans suffered from foot problems" (page 21) and suggests proper foot placement for balance and posture alignment (chapter 8, pages 71-74).

Sobel, D. and Klen, A. *Arthritis: What Exercises Work.* St Martin's Griffin. New York. 1993.

Sova, Ruth. *Water Fitness After 40.* Human Kinetics. Champaign. Illinois. 1995.

Page, Phil, and Ellenbecker, Todd. *Strength Band Training.* Human Kinetics. Champaign. Illinois. 1967.

Various Authors. *AKWA Magazine: The Official Publication of the Aquatic Exercise Association.* Nokomis. Florida. 1990-2012.

www.arthritis.org/exercise-intro.php. Arthritis Foundation Website

www.heart.org. American Heart Association Website

www.nih.gov./sites. National Institute of Health

http://www.naims.hih.gov. National Institute of Arthritis and Musculoskeletal and Skin Disease

www.mayoclinic.com/health/arthritis/ARC0030 *Hand Exercises for people with Arthritis*

www.everydayhealth.com/theumatoid-arthritis/6. Vann, Ph. D.M. Medically reviewed by Marcellinm M.D. M.PhD, L. *Six Hand Exercises for People with Rheumatoid Arthritis*

www.ehow.com. *How to Stretch Wrists, Hands, Fingers*

About the Author

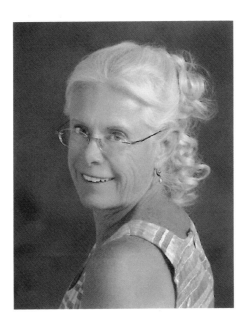

Born in the rural town of Tehachapi, California, Marti C. Sprinkle is a certified water aerobics instructor with over 25 years of experience. She is certified by the American Exercise Association and is also a member of the Aquatic Therapy and Rehabilitation Institute. She holds specialty certificates for Total Joint Replacement, Hip and Back, Integrated Core Training, and Rheumatology. For the past seven years Marti has specialized in therapeutic exercises in a commercial spa. She teaches water aerobics for all ages.

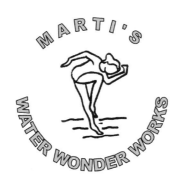

CPSIA information can be obtained
at www.ICGtesting.com
Printed in the USA
BVIC01n0358030114
340709BV00006B/94